Blood Analysis of Performance Horses

AND THE ROLE OF VITAMINS AND MINERALS

H D SHANNON
Assoc. Dip. Ag. (Equine)

MAX A HARRELL

First published 1994

Max A Harrell
4/444 Swan Street
Richmond Victoria 3121 Australia

National Library of Australia
Cataloguing-in-Publication data

Shannon, Henry D.
Blood analysis of performance horses and the role of vitamins and minerals.

Bibliography
ISBN 0 646 17227 1.

1. Horses - Health. 2. Blood - Analysis. 3. Vitamins in animal nutrition.
4. Minerals in animal nutrition. I. Title.

636.108910185

Produced by The Booksmith
Typeset by Mackenzies
Printed in Australia by McPherson's Printing Group

Contents

Tables

Foreword

This book should find a place in the libraries of all horsemen and horsewomen who own or train performance horses.

It will provide a ready reference in the areas of blood analysis and a guide to the equine requirements for minerals and vitamins.

The comments on proprietary supplements offer excellent advice on what the buyer should look for in the market place.

As the fields covered in this book are not, as yet, exact sciences, plenty of scope is provided for discussion on the topics. Not everyone will agree with all the author's conclusions but good evidence is always provided for such opinions.

It is written in language not too technical, which all readers should appreciate.

Anne McConnell B.V.Sc.

Author's Note

In writing this book, I was particularly fortunate to receive the advice and professional comments of Dr Anne McConnell, an Australian equine practitioner of considerable experience and expertise in the field.

Dr McConnell's input has been invaluable and I am deeply indebted to her for her willing assistance.

I am also indebted to Jane Napier who so willingly allowed me to use three of her thoroughbreds for blood testing.

Harry Shannon

Introduction

The aim of this book is to set out the theory and practice of blood analysis in performance horses. It aims to simplify some of the more technical terminology and make it more understandable for the average horseman. However, it is not set out merely as a theoretical discourse. In order to see what actually occurs in the field, three thoroughbred racehorses were selected, at various stages in their training schedules, and routinely blood tested over a six-week period. The results, analysis and conclusions drawn from these tests will be fully discussed in this book. Incidentally, although these tests were carried out in Australia, the same pattern of results would apply to any warm-blooded equine anywhere in the world. There could be minor changes because of environmental influences, but generally speaking, changes would be minimal and of no particular significance.

The majority of horsemen and horsewomen worldwide are not professionally qualified in equine science. This is not to say of course that they are not skilled in the day-to-day care and training of their horses. Many have spent a lifetime learning their craft. However, in keeping with our huge advance in technology in recent years, science is now playing a rapidly increasing part in the care and training of horses. This is more noticeable in the thoroughbred and harness racing industries where huge sums of money are invested. Rewards for the skilled and competent can be extremely high. As in every other endeavour in life the more highly skilled we are, the greater our chances of success.

In recent years great emphasis has been placed on blood analysis in the performance horse. Many veterinary clinics around the world specialise in providing this service. Some even have their own laboratories and technicians to carry the service to its conclusion.

Unfortunately, when many horse managers are handed the results of the test on their particular horse, they have little or no idea what it signifies and their veterinary surgeon has to provide a basic explanation of the analysis. Veterinarians are generally busy people and it would be unreasonable to expect time-consuming lectures on blood analysis interpretation to every client. Wouldn't it be much better if the horse manager had a reasonable idea of what it's all about before he or she started?

Veterinary surgeons and laboratory technicians, like the rest of us, are human and they can make mistakes. The results may not always appear what they seem, or they may not always give us the information we are seeking. Sometimes the picture is misleading. There are also one or two myths which have emerged in the matter of blood testing, particularly in the field of thoroughbred racing.

We have all heard trainers state that they cannot understand why their horse ran so badly, because they had been assured that the blood count was excellent. Quite often there is no clinical reason why the horse did not perform on the day. However, a blood count taken, say, 24 hours after the disappointing effort may show up some irregularity, such as the onset of an infection. Unfortunately, there is a belief, widely promoted by some, that the magical blood test will tell you precisely how your horse is and its level of fitness.

I am particularly interested in statements that blood testing would clearly show whether or not a horse is racing fit and at its peak, from the point of view of purely athletic fitness. This should not be confused with general overall health. Later on in this book, the reader will be able to examine the results of tests done on three thoroughbred racehorses over a six-week period. These tests turned up some very interesting results in two areas in particular and the reader may form his or her own judgement as to whether blood testing is an absolute guide to racing fitness.

Never lose sight of the fact, despite all the wonders of science, that the horse is a living, breathing animal, each unique in its own way and each an individual, just as with human beings.

We humans have all experienced days when we didn't 'feel' quite up to it. We didn't feel ill, our appetites were not affected, we looked well but somehow or other it just wasn't our day and we did not address our tasks with our normal vigour. Almost certainly our blood counts would have fallen within the 'normal' parameters for a healthy person. There is absolutely no reason to believe that a performance horse would react much differently. Everything seemed fine on the day, science said the blood count was fine, but the horse just didn't 'feel' like performing. The blood count will show that the horse is healthy and its red cell count may indicate that it is apparently fit, when taken into account with the other blood values. However it does not and never can guarantee that it will perform well on the day.

Blood testing is simply another tool of the trade of a competent horse manager and should be regarded as such only. The 'eye' of the experienced horsemanager will always be an excellent guide as to his or her horse's well-being. The horse will generally tell you itself when it is well and when it is fit. Experience will teach you these signs and it is not the purpose of this book to dwell at length on this aspect of horse care. Certainly, use blood testing as an occasional guide; it can be very valuable. It is particularly valuable, in fact almost essential, should you suspect that something is not quite right but that 'something' is not definable to your practised eye. Once again, the horse will tell you itself if it is not well; a blood test will confirm it. When correctly interpreted, it will also narrow down the field of diagnosis for you. Always regard blood testing as an excellent guide to general health but be just a little wary of its value as an inviolate indicator of racing fitness. That is not to say that it should be disregarded in this area. It has a value but don't lay too great a store by it.

When assessing the overall health and fitness of your horse, say, the evening before it runs, don't overlook resting pulse rate and respiration. They too are guides to fitness and well-being and they don't cost nearly as much as blood tests!

Remember also, that if you should have ten children, they will all be different. If you are training ten horses, so too will they be individually different. If you train and feed each one in precisely the same way, then unfortunately you will certainly not be regarded as a professional. It is also worth remembering that blood, because it is part of life and an integral component of a living body, is in a constant state of chemical and physical change. If you had your horse's blood count done at, say, 4pm on the day before a race, you will naturally receive a report showing certain values for that particular state of affairs at 4pm.

Should you take another sample at, say, 11am the following morning, then some of those values may be different. Admittedly, if your horse remained healthy overnight, they may not be markedly different and they will probably remain within acceptable limits but, rest assured, different they will be!

If you are a professional in the true sense of the word and you have taken the time to learn a little physiology, a little anatomy and a little chemistry along the way, you will soon get to know what the healthy, fit blood profile of each particular horse should be.

Hopefully after you have read this book and taken time out to study its contents, you will be fairly competent in understanding what the results of these tests actually mean. You will no longer have to take it on trust alone, on the word of someone else that all is well. You will also be able to take the appropriate remedial steps, if necessary with the assistance of your veterinary surgeon, should those results ring any alarm bells.

As a trainer, you have a very direct and very decisive input into what results your blood testing delivers. There are six important factors which directly determine the physical and physiological condition of your horse. They are *genetics, environment, nutrition, work regime, health care* and *handling*. As the trainer you have a very positive input into the end product; the only one you cannot influence is the genetic factor.

Therefore, to a very significant extent the result of your blood test will be the result of your professionalism in preparing your horse. Blood testing in horses is undertaken for two reasons — to reveal its health status and as a guide to its level of athletic fitness. Unlike humans, a horse is a natural athlete, which is no doubt a product of its evolution. Fitness, in a horse's natural open environment, meant that at all times it had to be ready to move quickly and to cover distance rapidly. When you check your horse's resting heart rate, you may be surprised to discover that the rate does not drop more than a few beats when it is race fit. On the other hand, a human athlete in good health will have a markedly decreased resting pulse rate when he or she has reached peak fitness. In spite of claims that blood testing will tell you when your horse is ready to win, the thoroughbred blood profile does not differ markedly between a fit healthy horse and a healthy horse which is nowhere near race fit.

It should be noted that for the purposes of this book we are talking about performance horses, Arabs, Quarter Horses, Thoroughbreds and Standardbreds. For want of a better description we may call the latter group 'Hot-blooded'. Ponies, draught horses and the like we may refer to as 'Cold-blooded'. There is some difference in the two, in respect to their red blood cells. Hot-bloods have more numerous but smaller red blood cells, whereas Cold-bloods have larger cells but a lower number. There are also other minor differences but we need not address ourselves to these at this time.

Blood Analysis

Let us now examine in some detail the more scientific aspects of this incredible substance we call blood and learn where its various components fit into the jigsaw.

Blood has been called the 'seat of the soul' because it bathes the body's tissues with fluids essential for support of life. Some of the major blood functions are as follows:

1 Transport of nutrients from the alimentary track to tissues.
2 Removal of waste products of metabolism.
3 Transport of oxygen to the tissues.
4 Transport of endocrine (glandular) secretions.
5 Equalisation of water content.
6 Temperature regulation.
7 Regulation of body acidity.
8 Defence against micro-organisms.
9 Immunity to disease.
10 Allergic reactions.

Blood is approximately 40% blood cells (corpuscles) and 60% carrying liquid (plasma). This plasma in itself carries protein, enzymes and electrolytes.

These cells are divided into three categories:
Red cells, *white* cells and *platelets* (clotting agents).

Red cells contain Haemoglobin (which gives blood its red colour). Haemoglobin is the carrier of oxygen around the body.

White blood cells (leucocytes) are the 'policemen' of the body.

TABLE 1   Haematology

UNIT	NORMAL LEVEL	POSSIBLE PROBLEMS IN ABNORMAL RESULTS	
Red Blood Cells (RBC) $\times 10^{12}$/L	8–11	Below 8.0	Worm infestation red worms; blood sucking varieties (internal) including heavy lice. External parasites. Protein deficiency and/or deficiency of iron, cobalt, copper, some B group vitamins. Impaired dietary efficiency. Destruction of red cells. Inability of bone marrow to replace red cells due to bone marrow suppression.
		Above 11.0	Dehydration, shock, excitement, exercise.
Haemoglobin (Hb) g/L	80–190 (Thoroughbred Arab etc 100–190)	Below 80	Anaemia, generally speaking the red cell count and Haemoglobin can be taken in conjunction.
Packed Cell Volume (PCV) L/L	0.30–0.47 (red cell to plasma ratio)	Below .30	Anaemia, worms, bone marrow problem. Broadly similar to RBC and Hb deficiency.
		Above .47	Dehydration, shock, excitement.

TABLE 1   Haematology (continued)

UNIT	NORMAL LEVEL	POSSIBLE PROBLEMS IN ABNORMAL RESULTS	
Mean Cell Corpuscular Volume (MCV) f L	41–49	Below 41	Iron deficiency, possible copper, cobalt, B group vitamin deficiency.
		Above 49	Possible increase of marrow activity responding to red cell destruction or haemorrhage.
Mean Corpuscular Haemoglobin (MCH) pg	13–16	Broadly similar remarks to values of RBC, Hb, PCV and MCV.	
Mean Corpuscular Haemoglobin Concentration (MCHC) g/L	30–36	Broadly similar remarks to values of RBC, Hb, PCV and MCV.	

They respond to injury, infection, allergies, stress and immune reaction. Blood testing is an extremely tedious, detailed and complicated procedure. Even the analysis of the results require some specialist training. Blood analysis is divided into three separate categories, Biochemistry, Microbiology and Haematology.

Biochemistry As the name implies, involves the examination of the blood chemistry. Biochemistry alone can encompass numerous separate tests. The important ones, as far as the performance horse is concerned, would be electrolytes, enzymes and proteins.

Microbiology Detection of organisms in the blood (through blood culture). The establishment of resistance or sensitivity to given antibiotics to be used in the treatment of such detected organisms often will not detect micro-organisms in blood, following acute state of infection. Therefore rising antibody titres may be useful to examine, eg two titres one month apart.

Haematology This covers the complete Red Cell, White Cell and Platelet constituents in the blood. These will be detailed as follows:

- Haemoglobin: (1g of Hb *can* bind with approximately 1.34 ml of oxygen)
- Red Cell Count: (RCC)
- Packed Cell Volume: (PCV) (Red Cell to Plasma ratio)
- Mean Corpuscular Volume: (MCV)
- Mean Corpuscular Haemoglobin: (MCH)
- Mean Corpuscular Haemoglobin Concentration (MCHC)
- Total White Cells: (Leucocytes) (WCC)
- Neutrophils
- Basophils
- Eosinophils
- Lymphocytes
- Monocytes
- Platelets

Even a casual perusal of these three categories of blood test procedures shows what an immense fund of information can be made available. A White Cell response to, say, stress, or viral infection (Haematology). An Enzyme analysis, say, CPK, for suspected muscle damage (Biochemistry).

For a blood count to be of real value we must know:

- Exactly what we require.
- How to interpret the result.
- What action to take, or if any action is necessary.

Tables are included showing the break-up of both the Haematology and Biochemistry Analysis in a typical equine profile. Against each Unit Hb, RBC, PCV etc are comments on possible reasons why that particular count may fall outside the norm.

When analysing the blood of a typical performance horse, we must decide what particular units we wish to examine. Having regard to numerous authorities and papers written by many researchers on the subject the following appears to be the typical equine profile:

Haematology   Haemoglobin (Hb)
       Red Cell Count (RCC)
       Packed Cell Volume (PCV or HCT)
       Mean Corpuscular Volume (MCV)
       Mean Corpuscular Haemoglobin (MCH)
       Mean Corpuscular Haemoglobin
        Concentration (MCHC)
       Total White Cells (Leucocytes) (WCC)
       Neutrophils
       Basophils
       Eosinophils
       Lymphocytes
       Monocytes

Biochemistry   Total Plasma Protein

$$\text{(TPP)} \left\{ \begin{array}{l} \text{Albumin} \\ \text{Globulin} \end{array} \right\} \text{A:G ratio}$$

       Sodium (Na)
       Potassium (K)
       Chloride (Cl)
       Enzymes: Creatinine Phospho Kinase (CPK)

> Aspartate Trans Aminase (AST)
> Alkaline Phosphatase
> Gamma GT
> Inorganic Phosphate
> Bilirubin.

If each one of these readings falls within the parameters of the *normal* values, then probably we have a very healthy horse. However the 'bottom line' of blood testing today seems to be whether or not our horse is *100% fit to win*. It seems to be often overlooked that *HEALTH* and *FITNESS* are *not* the same thing. Obviously a fit horse *must* be healthy. Note: These parameters *may* still be normal in certain disease processes or with some injuries.

However, a perfectly healthy horse may not necessarily be fit. For example a horse which is still in the paddock after six weeks spelling may be healthy but certainly not race fit.

Now we shall examine these components in a little more detail.

Haemoglobin (HB)   Haemoglobin accounts for the bright red colour of blood. It is usually expressed in grams per litre of blood. It is manufactured by cells in the bone marrow. Elements such as iron, copper, cobalt are necessary for its manufacture, as is protein. It follows that any serious deficiencies in these elements would have a serious effect. The iron from haemoglobin is stored in the liver, spleen and kidneys.

Red Cells   These contain the haemoglobin and are responsible for the transport of oxygen around the body. In theory, at least, a high average Red Cell count should indicate fitness and the ability of the cardiovascular system of the horse to supply large amounts of oxygen to the hard-working tissues.

Packed Cell Volume (PCV)   This is an indication of the ratio of cellular constituents to the total volume of blood.

Mean Cell Volume (MCV), **Mean Cell Haemoglobin**(MCH), **Mean Cell Haemoglobin Concentration** (MCHC) These three are not actual tests of measurement but they are a calculation involving Packed Cell Volume (PCV), Red Blood Cell Count (RBCC) and Haemoglobin percentage.

White Cells These are collectively termed *leucocytes* and can be collectively or bulk measured in an analysis. However, they are divided into specific cells as follows:

Neutrophils These are the most abundant of the white cells. They act as front line defence in the onset of infection. They are attracted to the immediate site of inflammation and their purpose is to overwhelm the foreign bodies.

Basophils These cells contain the hormone histamine, which acts to dilate blood vessels to allow a greater volume of healing blood to an injured area. They also act in the blood in such a way as to aid the migration of neutrophils to the problem area.

Eosinophils They control the extent of inflammation at the site of the injury. In other words they provide a counter balance to de-activate histamine and inflammatory reactions.

Lymphocytes These can be seen as small and large lymphocytes. The large ones stored in the lymph nodes act as a barrier to germs entering the body. Small lymphocytes continuously circulate in the blood and they have the ability to detect or recognise previously neutralised germs. They have an antibody function. It is extremely complex and the above is a very simplified explanation.

Monocytes These are large cells and generally small in number in the healthy equine. They, like most white cells, multiply during times of infection. They act similarly to neutrophils and they have had a hand in the production of antibodies. As far as this book is concerned, the biochemistry aspect has been confined to *Plasma protein, Sodium (Na), Potassium (K), Chloride (Cl)* and three enzymes.

Creatinine Phospho Kinase (CPK), **Aspartate Trans Aminase** (AST), **Alkaline Phosphatase** (ALP) Refer to result tables for remarks, as to specific observations for these particular enzymes. Most researchers and authorities seem to broadly agree that these represent the important components as far as blood analysis in the performance horse is concerned. By the way, enzymes are technically described, in general terms, as

TABLE 2   **White Cell Count**

UNIT	NORMAL LEVEL	POSSIBLE PROBLEMS IN ABNORMAL RESULTS	
Total white blood cells leucocytes (WBC) 10^9/L	6.5–12.0	Below 6.5	Overwhelming bacterial infections. Long-term stress and/or prolonged hard training. Long-term use of antibiotics. Long-term use of anti inflammatory drugs.
		Above 12.0	Moderate to serious infections depending upon level. Leukaemia. Body's allergic response to skin infections and/or parasites. Possible elevation could result from exercise prior to blood collection or excitement. Early stress response can cause increased WBC count.
Neutrophils (N) 10^9/L	2.4–6.7	Below 2.4 Above 6.7	Overwhelming bacterial infection. (Neutrophilia) surgery, injury, severe internal haemorrhage. Tissue damage. Long-term stress. Infection.
Basophils (B) 10^9/L	0–0.36	Above 0.36	Serious liver damage possibly due to toxins, e.g. ingestion of toxic plants such as Paterson's Curse.

TABLE 2   White Cell Count (continued)

UNIT	NORMAL LEVEL	POSSIBLE PROBLEMS IN ABNORMAL RESULTS	
Eosinophils (E) 10^9/L	0.6–0.9	Below 0.6	Inflammation, injury, infection, overtraining, stress. Anti-inflammatory drug administration.
		Above 0.9	Inflammatory response. Allergic reactions. Internal parasites.
Lymphocytes (L) 10^9/L	1.6–5.4	Below 1.6	Long-term stress. Anti-inflammatory drug treatment (ie corticosteroids).
		Above 5.4	Convalescence from severe illness. Chronic infection. Severe malnutrition. Leukaemia.
Monocytes (M) 10^9/L	0–0.36	Above 0.36	Can show in recovery phase from infections and/or tissue damage.

being a protein catalyst of a specific biochemical reaction in the body. It is most interesting to note that almost all the 'blood story' aspects for the horse apply to human beings, in almost exactly the same way.

Note: Significance of raised enzyme levels in the blood lies in the fact that certain body cells have to be damaged for the enzymes to escape into the circulation, eg muscle cell → AST, CPK, epithelial cells → ALP.

We have now identified the various blood constituents that we wish to examine in the horse. Tables 1, 2 and 3 show what authorities deem to be 'average' healthy levels of each constituent under examination and what departure from these norms may be telling us.

Naturally it must be appreciated that these 'normal' levels have been arrived at over time by researchers worldwide. They can never be absolute and they will vary in individuals, sometimes quite markedly without any apparent effect on a particular horse. As far as stressed performance horses are concerned, some authorities might regard these normal ranges as being too broad.

It may be readily observed that haematology is really all about Red Blood Cell Count and Haemoglobin levels. White blood cells and platelets PCV, MCV and MCHC counts are totally inter-related. However, departures from normal levels of all or any of these six factors generally point to the same problems, and for the purposes of this exercise there is no need to become too immersed in the technicalities of these six components.

Another very important point which should be stressed here is the meaning and use of the word *anaemia*. It would be fair to say that the majority of people believe anaemia to be a disease, or an illness, in itself. This is not the case; it is a symptom and has many causes. Again, most of us associate anaemia with iron deficiency in the body, the simple cure being supplementation by an iron tonic. Broadly speaking the anaemic condition is brought about by the depletion and/or destruction of red cells and we have to investigate why this may be so. In the case of the

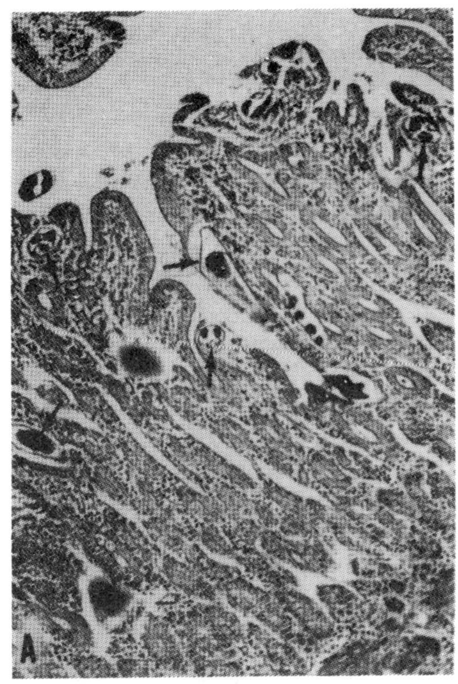

Strongyloidosis (Strongyloides weteri), small intestine of colt (x 75). Numerous small immature worms (see arrows) burrowing in mucosa.

equine, the most likely cause of moderate to severe anaemia revealed by an RBC and Hb count would be due to red worm infestation. Provided we are not too late, your veterinary surgeon will advise what action may be taken to solve the problem.

Remember that in a healthy horse enjoying a prime quality balanced diet, iron deficiency is highly unlikely. Generally speaking the well-managed horse always has iron excess to its requirements and iron-rich commercial blood tonic supplements are unnecessary.

It can be observed that there are many common denominators in the various constituent components of White Blood Cells and abnormality in any one of these can often point to the same illness. Overall, therefore, it is obvious that in general terms the White Cell Count is the most important factor.

Whilst still on the subject of White Cells some research points

TABLE 3   Biochemistry

UNIT	NORMAL LEVEL	POSSIBLE PROBLEMS IN ABNORMAL RESULTS	
Total protein g/L	53–76	Below 53	Low protein, malnutrition, poor appetite, poor feeder. Internal parasites, protein loss. Diarrhoea. Haemorrhage. Liver disease. Last 3 months of pregnancy and also during lactation. Stress.
		Above 76	Dehydration. Increased production of globulin. Advancing age.
Sodium (Na) mmol/L	135–144	Below 135	Parasites, bacterial changes in the gut. Bad diarrhoea. Chronic renal failure. Water excess.
		Above 144	Dehydration. Not eating or drinking. Water deprivation. Acute general infection. Look for dull coat, dull eyes. Slow skin return to pinch test (which is a sign of dehydration, not necessarily low Na).

TABLE 3   Biochemistry (continued)

UNIT	NORMAL LEVEL	POSSIBLE PROBLEMS IN ABNORMAL RESULTS	
Potassium (K) mmo/L	3.4–4.2	Below 3.4	Heavy sweat loss. Increased urine excretion, excessive use of kidney tonics. Excessive use of mineralocorticoid drugs which increase K excretion while retaining Na. (Diarrhoea depletes K to a lesser extent than Na.) Plasma K levels are critical for survival because of the effects on cardiac and neuromuscular functions.
		Above 4.2	Severe injury. Long-term stress. Acidosis. Acute renal failure (also caused artificially due to blood being stored too long before analysis).
Chlorides (Cl) mmol/L	96–103	Below 96	Excessive sweat loss. Alkalosis.
		Above 103	Dehydration, diarrhoea, acidosis.

TABLE 3 Biochemistry (continued) – selected enzymes

Creatinine Phospho Kinase (CPK) IU/L	* Less than 100	Elevated CPK. Heart, skeletal muscle damage (tying up, heart strain).
Aspartate Trans Aminase (AST) IU/L	* Less than 400	Elevated AST. Same as CPK but with the addition of liver damage. Drug induced causes. Transient exercise induced rises. Particularly skeletal muscle damage. Gut damage, eg gastro enteritis. General cell leakage.
Alkaline Phosphatase (ALP) IU/L	* Less than 180	Elevated ALP. Liver disease, inflammatory obstruction to bile flow. Bone diseases (can show up also in bone healing). Can be elevated during pregnancy. Skin diseases. Parasites. Drug induced rises. Normally higher in young horse due to bone growth.

* Many experienced practitioners would see these levels as too low in performance horses. This view is borne out by the results obtained in our tests.

to the diagnostic usefulness of neutrophil to lymphocyte ratio (N/L). It has been shown that an immediate response to the stress or anticipation of exercise results in an increase of lymphocytes, with a decrease in the N/L ratio. How significant this may be is open to opinion but it is an interesting observation. Ratio may be in the order of 1.5:1. Long-term stress of training can result in N/L reversal.

The CPK and AST enzymes are sometimes referred to as the muscle enzymes. Numerous tests and experiments have often shown significant rises in these levels resulting from muscle damage and/or 'tying up' (build up of lactic acid in muscle tissue, often following hard exercise).

However, we shall see later in this book that this theory, in particular, did not reinforce itself in our field tests over the six-week period. Before proceeding to the description of the subjects of the field tests we shall examine the mechanics of the actual blood collection.

Collection procedure and equipment

Having selected the laboratory which will be doing your blood analysis, obtain from them the blood collection tubes. They will supply them to you at no charge. (Incidentally, I would tend to discourage untrained operators from carrying out their own sampling and testing. This role is better left to experienced veterinary practitioners.) You will require *two* tubes for each sample. This is because the lab requires blood in two forms. The first form is *WHOLE* blood for the Haematology section and *SERUM* for the Biochemistry section.

If the blood is allowed to stand for even a short time it will start to settle and divide. The Red Blood Cells, the most numerous (this is the packed cell volume), will congeal and the remaining separated clear liquid is the serum. Fluid left after blood clotting is *SERUM*; fluid left after blood is spun down is *PLASMA* (ie blood collected with anti-coagulant). The serum will be analysed to reveal the protein, enzymes and electrolytes. Between the RBCs and the plasma is the narrow layer ('buffy coat') containing the total white cells (much less numerous than the red cells in number).

During the time between actually collecting the sample and the delivery to the lab, the blood would have congealed. As a result the analysis of the red and white cells would be impossible as they would have coagulated. The lab will therefore give you a special tube which contains an *anti-coagulant*. This will stop the blood from clotting in this particular tube.

You will therefore have the two tubes for collections, as mentioned: one small tube for the whole blood and one larger tube for the serum (clotted blood). These are clearly marked by the manufacturers and generally colour coded as well.

You will see a specific graduation mark on the whole blood tube. It will probably be either 2.5 ml or 5 ml. The tube *MUST* be filled to this mark, neither more nor less. This is important as the anti-coagulant material in the tube is a measured quantity which is matched to the amount of blood specified on the label.

The amount of blood collected in the serum tube is not critical. Approximately 10 ml plus would be sufficient for most labs in the serum tube. Syringe size is not critical but it should be at least 20 ml capacity. My own experience is that 20 cc is a good all-round size because you may find that you wish to give the *same* blood sample to different labs for comparison purposes. Needle size is much more critical. Gauge should be 18 or 19 and length 38 mm.

The method of collection is quite straightforward and it is surprising how proficient one becomes with just a little practice. It is recommended that a horse with placid disposition is used for one's first attempt.

The most convenient site for collection is the near side jugular vein, approximately two-thirds up the neck from the point of the shoulder. The vein is easily located in the jugular furrow on the neck. Firstly distend the vein by firm left thumb pressure on the vein approximately 30 cm from the point of the shoulder. This will block the venous blood flow down the vein and naturally cause it to swell or distend above the thumb pressure. Next tap the distended vein with your free hand and both feel and observe the blood movement in the vein. This is quite important because the jugular vein is quite large, approximately the size of one's third finger, when distended. It can be confused with muscle in this neck area but by tapping the vein and 'feeling' the blood movement, a mistake should not be made.

Having identified and distended the vein, you may now insert the needle with the free right hand. It is vital to keep the vein distended whilst inserting the needle. Position the needle at approximately 45° to the skin with the bevelled edge facing to the skin to aid easy penetration.

Next with firm and positive pressure push the needle through into the vein. As soon as you have penetrated the skin and vein approximately to a depth of one cm up the needle, immediately change your needle angle and run the remainder of the needle flat to the horse's neck and directly up into and parallel with the distended vein.

You will note that blood will flow fairly quickly, provided you have punctured the vein correctly and provided you keep the vein distended.

Next insert your collection syringe onto your inserted needle and slowly withdraw the required volume of blood. (Vacuutainer tubes may also be used.)

Occasionally the blood flow may appear too slow or stop; if so gently move the syringe around quietly in the vein. This will restore the flow. It is *essential* to keep the thumb pressure on the vein during extraction of the blood. When filled, remove the syringe and needle gently but positively. The vein will seal itself almost instantly.

It is common practice for the operator to first clean the skin, with a solution of either alcohol or methylated spirits. (This procedure is more for the benefit of the owner and onlooker, rather than the horse.) Ostensibly it may seem to thoroughly clean the area and render it sterile. In practice such a cursory cleaning cannot achieve this effect. Provided the neck is free from any obvious dirt or soiling, you may simply insert your needle without this cosmetic cleaning technique. There is one very obvious disadvantage of using a cleaning agent first, and that is the odour. Most horses are very sensitive to smell, and the strong smell of such liquids invariably alerts an otherwise relaxed horse that something rather nasty is about to take place, certainly something beyond normal daily routine handling.

It is of course of *vital* importance that a *sterile* needle *and* syringe is used for each and every sampling. Any contamination in either can be very dangerous, as far as introducing an infection to a horse. It can also totally ruin the collected blood, rendering the analysis useless.

Immediately the syringe has been withdrawn detach the needle and place the blood in each of the two sampling container tubes, firstly into the tube with anti-coagulant. Press the syringe plunger *slowly*, as it is possible to rupture blood cells in the process, causing cell leakage in the sample. This will severely affect its correct analysis. *Never* place the blood in the containers through the needle; this will increase the pressure greatly, favouring cell rupture.

In regard to the whole blood sample, it is important to ensure good and quick mixing in the tube with the anti-coagulant. Rotate the tube gently to achieve this; *don't* shake as this will tend to rupture cells also.

The blood should then be delivered to the lab as soon as possible, preferably within 2–3 hours. It is *not* recommended to keep it overnight under refrigeration. Blood cells can be damaged if chilled below 4°C. Expansion could result in cell wall damage and leakage of cell contents, giving false readings. It is generally sufficient to wrap the tubes in cotton wool or tissues and then place them in a foam drink container, or similar. Some pathologists prefer the blood at room temperature, as chilling can damage the cells, as mentioned above.

Cell walls start to deteriorate after six hours and may leak electrolytes. This is why it is not recommended to keep blood overnight. Don't forget to clearly mark each container with the horse's name and date and time of sampling.

For the purpose of our six-week field testing, three thorough-bred racehorses were selected.

Horse 1: two-year-old filly
Horse 2: three-year-old filly
Horse 3: four-year-old mare.

It should be noted that sex is irrelevant in the matter of blood analysis. It was coincidental that the three horses chosen were in fact female. They were selected mainly because they were in varying stages of training, also their temperaments were different. The age grouping was deliberate because I wanted to see whether any marked difference could be noticed because of the age factor. As it turned out nothing was observed in the various blood counts which indicated that age had any significant effect.

Sampling was commenced on a specific day and continued at exactly seven-day intervals for six weeks. On average, samples were taken at around 11 am each morning, which allowed the animals to recover from early morning exercise, which took place generally between the hours of 6–8 am. Therefore, each horse had between three–five hours to relax before blood was taken. It is important, when blood is being taken, that the horse is at rest and as relaxed as possible. Blood of course is often deliberately taken immediately after strenuous exercise. However, this is done with a very specific aim in mind and is not the subject of this book.

The resting period referred to assists the blood status to return to normal and allows for stabilisation of Red Cells, Electrolytes and packed cell volume in particular. Samples were taken strictly in accordance with the procedures previously outlined and the blood was delivered fresh to the laboratory, generally within two hours of being taken.

Many practitioners feel that the most consistent results come from sampling before the horse leaves the stable in the morning, otherwise approximately six hours post-work, which we did in our sampling.

The status of the three horses at the commencement of the experiment was as follows:

The two-year-old had just come into training and had commenced very light exercise, walking, trotting and jogging.

The three-year-old had been in work six weeks and judged by her trainer as about three-parts fit at this stage. Generally she was regarded as a 'poor doer' but otherwise reasonably easy to handle and train. Her temperament was good, as was the two-year-old's.

The four-year-old had been eight weeks in work and was approaching racing fitness. She ran on two occasions during the six-week sampling period and trialled once. She acquitted herself creditably on each occasion and her trainer was reasonably pleased. She then ran some days after the final sample was taken and on that occasion ran a very good fourth in a metropolitan race. It would be fair to say that she would have been at peak racing fitness at the time of the last sampling. Of the three subjects she was the most difficult. She tended to be highly strung, on occasions difficult to handle and always a heavy sweater. She was therefore a very interesting subject for comparison with the other two.

Neither of the other two ran during the sampling period. However the three-year-old ran for the first time two weeks after the last sample and she won comfortably at a metropolitan meeting.

Following is the analysis for each horse, showing the results obtained over the six weeks.

Results of analysis over six weeks

Bear in mind the experiment was conducted to compare any changes which might occur over a six-week training programme and to investigate whether any conclusion could be arrived at to enable assessment of racing fitness. All horses were clinically healthy at the commencement and happily their health and well-being was retained during the period.

It was not expected therefore that any marked deviation from the norm would be observed in the leucocytes. The results show this to be the case. There was one minor increase in eosinophils, in the two-year-old. It was back to normal however the following week. The trainer did report, interestingly enough, that the filly had developed a slight cold for a few days during that time. However, it should be noted that this would not be the normal eosinophil response expected in such circumstances. Eosinophils usually decrease with stress. However, with certain viral infections, eosinophil levels may be raised.

It will be noted that in week three, there was a dramatic drop in the two-year-old's haemoglobin (Hb) and red cell count (RCC). The filly was immediately examined but found to be in perfect health and normal high spirits. The laboratory claimed that their figures were correct. However, in the light of some interesting comparative figures, which shall be included at the conclusion of the book, one wonders! With the one exception mentioned above the haematology results were virtually 'average' over the period for all three subjects.

It has been generally accepted that the Hb and RCC will tend to follow an upward movement as a horse progresses to full fitness. Naturally it will vary from individual to individual.

This has been confirmed by the experiment, to some extent. These rises, however, were neither dramatic nor uniform. It is particularly noticeable that the final counts were actually *lower* in the four-year-old and three-year-old, than some previous counts. It is particularly significant that both horses either won or ran very well at the end of the period. The inevitable conclusion must be that there was no significant rise in either Hb or RCC when these horses reached peak fitness.

There is a much cherished and long-held belief amongst researchers that excitement and nervousness will result in artificially inflated Hb and RCC. It is believed that the 'spenic response' of a nervous horse at sampling will result in a veritable rush of red cells into the blood-stream. This was certainly *NOT* shown to be the case with any of these horses.

The two-year-old was very placid and virtually couldn't have cared less whether you were sticking needles in her or not.

The three-year-old became a little agitated, but quite manageable, although her heart rate generally increased.

However, the four-year-old mare was *always* highly excitable and always strongly resisted the sampling. On one occasion, she was so fractious that it was impossible to continue. The trainer finally calmed her sufficiently and she took the sample from the horse herself after much ado.

It was extremely significant that there was no noticeable rise in RCC on that occasion. After 18 samplings, the only conclusion that can possibly be reached is that the so-called 'nervous splenic response' is grossly exaggerated. However, if a given horse was always excitable, it is possible that its RCC could always be elevated, for that particular horse. The splenic response could also have been a factor.

We now come to what appears to be the most significant part of the exercise, which appears in the biochemistry. The electrolytes were normal throughout the experiment with the exception of potassium in the four-year-old, at the first sampling. (Remember this is a heavy sweater.) On enquiry, the trainer advised that the mare had bolted with her rider that morning and of course had lost even more sweat than usual.

As a result, we experimented by substituting potassium chloride for sodium chloride, in her diet. The following week her K level returned to normal and remained normal despite her heavy work load and two races in between.

The real puzzle has been the enzyme results.

As we can see from the biochemistry interpretation tables (Table 3), elevated CPK, AST and ALP levels are associated with such problems as muscle damage, heart strain, bone disease, liver disease, skin disease, internal parasites, and drug-induced elevation. CPK elevation, for example, is regarded as the typical 'tying up' pointer.

On examination of all three enzyme counts in *each* horse over the six weeks it can be seen that all enzymes were elevated on most occasions, in many instances some ten times or more 'average' levels.

All horses were immediately checked but were found to be clinically in perfect health. Their endeavours on the racecourse prove the point. At no time did any of the horses tie up nor did they show even minor stiffness or discomfort. Parasite control in the stable was good and no drugs were being administered during the period.

The attention of the laboratory was drawn to these high and dramatically fluctuating figures. They responded by saying that they would stand by their results and that their technique was beyond doubt.

The 'normal ranges' shown on the result sheets were arrived at by figures quoted by most researchers and text books. It is very difficult therefore to come to any worthwhile conclusion as far as the significance of enzyme counts are concerned.

One is forced to conclude that the 'normal ranges' are set far too low as far as thoroughbreds are concerned, either that or elevated enzymes are not of great significance and do not have much bearing on the health or fitness state of the horse. Based on these experiments there is no other possible conclusion that one could reach. However, as we have noted earlier these enzyme 'normal' levels appear to be set too low for racehorses.

Rarely does one read, in text books or papers, any reference to the efficiency or expertise of the *laboratories* which do the actual blood testing.

With this in mind it was decided to compare *three* professional laboratories by submitting the *same* blood sample to each laboratory.

One full syringe sample was collected from the four-year-old and divided equally into three containers and delivered to the three laboratories. It was delivered fresh to all three within two hours.

A comparison of the results makes very interesting reading(see page 37). The three laboratories agreed on only three counts against 19 constituents analysed. Admittedly they were close enough in most areas for the results to be credible.

For obvious reasons the labs have not been named specifically and a lettercode A, B, C, is used to identify each one.

There was a dramatic difference in the RCC in which lab A showed a figure almost *one third* lower than the other two. Yet the HB, PCV and MCV almost agreed with the others. There must be some question mark against lab A in the area of RCC because on one occasion they failed to submit a figure claiming some problem with the equipment.

In all other areas, however, lab A agreed for the most part with lab C. The one that was out of step most often with the other two was lab B.

Summary of conclusions on the six-week experiment are as follows:

1 There is no dramatic rise in either Hb or RCC as the horse progresses towards racing fitness.
2 The splenic response from the nervous or excited horse is barely discernible. It can virtually be disregarded, if these results are to be believed.
3 Leucocyte levels remain markedly stable (which one would expect) in healthy horses and they show no discernible movement as the horse progresses towards racing fitness.
4 Plasma protein and electrolytes show practically no variation, the only solitary exception being low potassium in the heavy-sweating, stressed horse. This was easily corrected, as outlined.
5 The enzymes CPK, AST and ALP fluctuated violently. No clinical problems could be detected which might have explained this. All three horses remained healthy, bright and fit and were able to win or run extremely well in good city company.
6 Because of the enzyme results obtained, it is obvious that the 'normal' range has been set far too low by many researchers. It follows that not too much significance should be placed on high counts *unless* accompanied by some clinical signs of infection, or distress.
7 The actual results obtained by laboratories seem open to question on many occasions.

8 Blood testing is an excellent guide to health but questionable as an infallible guide to peak racing fitness.

It is hoped that the 'blood picture' will now be much easier for the reader to understand. In future, when you receive the result sheet from your horse's test, you will be able to understand more fully its health status and condition. It is a wonderful scientific tool, to be used wisely, and there are often important lessons to be learned. It is worth noting, when studying blood testing figures, the important role of drug administration in horses and indeed in humans also. It is clearly illustrated that excess drug therapy can have serious effects and will distort the blood profile dramatically. It can also have serious long-term effects on your horse. However, your veterinary surgeon will be the best judge of this aspect. I am more concerned with the disturbing modern trend of random unprofessional administration of drugs to horses, with a view to improving performance and/or masking the pain symptoms of serious problems. The latter is particularly prevalent in the case of anti-inflammatory drugs. Always remember, just as in humans, the golden rule must be — treat the problem not the symptom.

A comment on anabolic steroids is in order because these also will distort your blood picture. Steroids can and are successfully used by the veterinary profession in treating certain ailments in horses. Again your own vet will be the best judge of when these should be used. However, don't be fooled into thinking that an injection or two, on the side, will build up race-winning muscle on your horse. The genetics alone determine exactly how much muscle can be laid down on the skeleton. This rule applies to humans also.

Administration of anabolic steroids will certainly encourage premature muscle tissue build-up. However, it has some particularly damaging side-effects. Used in young horses, at least up to three years, it will add muscle weight to immature skeletons. Nature did not intend this to be so and the results will inevitably lead to bone, tendon and ligament damage.

In these early stages of skeletal development, nature did not intend them to carry this excess. Other functions may also suffer some trauma, such as the cardio-vascular system. One of the other inter-related side-effects is that anabolic steroids will give a false impression of muscle mass. They induce fluid build-up in the muscle tissue, which of course adds extra weight in itself. Being fluid, it is totally non-productive in the muscle and plays no part in muscle function, other than to add more weight for the skeleton to carry. Unfortunately there is a tendency for some stud farms to use steroids in yearlings, prior to sale. Certainly they look strong and heavily muscled but the results can be devastating as those yearlings are broken and put into work.

A few studs do this because there is an unfortunate tendency for some buyers to favour this sort of burly yearling presentation. Obviously those particular people have no knowledge of equine anatomy or physiology.

As may be seen from the tables in this book, uncontrolled steroid administration will show up in your blood tests and the systemic damage they cause may be irreversible, quite apart from skeletal trauma. As previously mentioned, notwithstanding the effects steroids appear to have, you cannot build additional muscle in excess of the limits imposed by the genetic composition of the individual.

If you allow your horse to mature and you employ a trained professional work programme, together with a scientifically balanced diet and healthy environment, your horse will reach its determined genetic potential in the fullness of time. Regrettably I cannot assure you that it will win when this theoretical summit has been reached but at least you will have given it every chance.

It is worth repeating that what has been enumerated in this book in no way claims to represent the complete science of blood analysis, many aspects of which have not been referred to at all. The parameters examined are those which most researchers agree are the important ones to analyse in assessing the health and fitness of the performing horse. Individual opinions obviously exist which would favour either the addition or subtraction of specific data.

Again some experienced researchers will be somewhat surprised by some of the results, particularly the enzymes. However, facts are facts and that is exactly how they came out, after every precaution was taken. The laboratories used are highly regarded and extensively patronised by both the veterinary and medical professions. The fact that they produced some differing results from identical samples is most interesting. Readers may draw their own conclusions.

Note: The following were *not* tested: inorganic phosphate, albumin: globulin ratio and GGT. However, the following comments may be useful.

Inorganic Phosphate: 0.90–1.65 range. Used as a meter of metabolism. Low level means no growth, poor anabolic rate. High levels means growth spurt. Probably more important to request this test in very young, growing horses.

Albumin: Globulin Ratio: Normally about 1:1. An alteration in favour of globulin can mean an infection. Should be interpreted in the light of WCC results.

GGT: A seldom requested enzyme test but some experienced practitioners feel that it can be important in some individuals. Elevation often points to incorrect training programme for that horse. Experience seems to indicate that a horse with a reading over 100 will not race well without a long spell in the paddock. Normal range is up to 38. Higher than this may point to stress in the training regime.

Table 4   Equine Blood Analysis   6-Week Period

Haematology 2-year-old filly	Unit	Normal Range	Week 1	Week 2	Week 3	Week 4	Week 5	Week 6
Haemoglobin (Hb)	g/L	110–160	127	130	77*	141	151	138
Red Cell Count (RCC)	10^{12}/L	7.5–11	6.61	6.76	3.89*	9.4	7.7	10.5
Packed Cell Volume (PCV) (HCT)	L/L	0.30–0.48	0.30	0.30	0.17	0.37	0.34	0.49
Mean Corpuscular Volume (MCV) (Red Cells)	fl	41–49	45.2	44.8	43.8	39	45	37
Mean Corpuscular Haemoglobin (MCH)	g/L	13–16	19.2	19.2	19.8	15	19.6	13
Mean Corpuscular Haemoglobin Concentration (MCHC)	g/L	300–360	425	429	452	380	436	360
Total White Cells (Leucocytes) (WCC)	10^9/L	6–12	9	10	2.8	8.8	10.1	10.2
Neutrophils	10^9/L	2–7	5.76	5.5	1.68	4.04	5.05	5.71
Basophils	10^9/L	0–0.3	Nil	Nil	Nil	Nil	Nil	Nil
Eosinophils	10^9/L	0.1–0.5	1.08	0.5	0.08	Nil	0.2	Nil
Lymphocytes	10^9/L	1.6–5.4	1.8	3.6	0.81	4.57	4.44	3.67
Monocytes	10^9/L	0.6–0.7	0.36	0.4	0.22	0.17	0.4	0.82
Biochemistry								
Total Plasma Protein (TPP)	g/L	53–76	64	63	63	61	65	67
Sodium (Na)	MMO/L	135–144	131	132	137	138	136	139
Potassium (K)	MMO/L	3.4–4.2	3.4	3.2	3	3.7	3.4	3.8
Chloride (Cl)	MMO/L	96–103	97	96	100	104	99	No result
Enzymes CPK (Creatinine Phospho Kinase)	U/L	< 100	165	222	328	100	2259	276
AST (Aspartate Trans Aminase)	U/L	< 400	277	280	313	208	401	339
ALP (Alkaline Phosphatase)	U/L	< 180	327	356	332	660	305	327

*Obviously, incorrect laboratory analysis.

Table 5   Equine Blood Analysis   6-Week Period

Haematology 3-year-old filly	Unit	Normal Range	Week 1	Week 2	Week 3	Week 4	Week 5	Week 6
Haemoglobin (Hb)	g/L	110–160	147	144	148	190	177	159
Red Cell Count (RCC)	10^{12}/L	7.5–11	7.82	7.66	7.85	12.7	No result	11.22
Packed Cell Volume (PCV) (HCT)	L/L	0.30–0.48	0.37	0.36	0.36	0.50	No result	0.46
Mean Corpuscular Volume (MCV) (Red Cells)	fl	41–49	47	46.8	46.6	39	47.3	41
Mean Corpuscular Haemoglobin (MCH)	g/L	13–16	18.8	18.8	18.9	15	No result	14
Mean Corpuscular Haemoglobin Concentration (MCHC)	g/L	300–360	400	402	405	380	No result	340
Total White Cells (Leucocytes) (WCC)	10^9/L	6–12	10.2	8.8	7.7	11.4	9.8	11
Neutrophils	10^9/L	2–7	5.71	4.75	3.38	6.38	5.29	5.28
Basophils	10^9/L	0–0.3	0.10	Nil	Nil	Nil	Nil	Nil
Eosinophils	10^9/L	0.1–0.5	0.3	0.17	0.15	Nil	0.19	Nil
Lymphocytes	10^9/L	1.6–5.4	3.67	3.52	3.85	5.01	3.92	5.5
Monocytes	10^9/L	0.6–0.7	0.4	0.35	0.30	Nil	0.39	0.22
Biochemistry								
Total Plasma Protein (TPP)	g/L	53–76	65	62	65	67	66	64
Sodium (Na)	MMO/L	135–144	130	135	135	138	135	139
Potassium (K)	MMO/L	3.4–4.2	3.9	2.7	3	3.9	3.2	3.2
Chloride (Cl)	MMO/L	96–103	98	97	99	98	100	No result
Enzymes CPK (Creatinine Phospho Kinase)	U/L	< 100	528	308	3474	407	475	1283
AST (Aspartate Trans Aminase)	U/L	< 400	593	554	1683	1147	718	527
ALP (Alkaline Phosphatase)	U/L	< 180	176	152	159	367	163	191

Table 6   **Equine Blood Analysis**   **6-Week Period**   **Date of 3 Lab Blood Comparisons**

Haematology 4-year-old mare	Unit	Normal Range	Week 1	Week 2	Week 3	Week 4	Week 5	Week 6
Haemoglobin (Hb)	g/L	110–160	172	153	173	171	183	161
Red Cell Count (RCC)	10^{12}/L	7.5–11	9.1	8.07	9.24	11.4	9.65	11.5
Packed Cell Volume (PCV) (HCT)	L/L	0.30–0.48	0.43	0.38	0.43	0.45	0.45	0.44
Mean Corpuscular Volume (MCV) (Red Cells)	fl	41–49	46.7	46.6	46.5	39	47	39
Mean Corpuscular Haemoglobin (MCH)	g/L	13–16	18.9	19	18.7	15	19	14
Mean Corpuscular Haemoglobin Concentration (MCHC)	g/L	300–360	405	407	403	380	400	360
Total White Cells (Leucocytes) (WCC)	10^9/L	6–12	10	8.4	9.8	7.6	9.1	10
Neutrophils	10^9/L	2–7	6	4.53	8.23	5.77	5.09	6
Basophils	10^9/L	0–0.3	Nil	0.08	Nil	Nil	Nil	Nil
Eosinophils	10^9/L	0.1–0.5	0.05	0.16	0.09	Nil	0.18	0.2
Lymphocytes	10^9/L	1.6–5.4	2.8	2.94	1.37	1.82	3.64	3.7
Monocytes	10^9/L	0.6–0.7	0.7	0.67	0.09	Nil	0.18	0.10
Biochemistry								
Total Plasma Protein (TPP)	g/L	53–76	63	60	60	59	61	58
Sodium (Na)	MMO/L	135–144	130	136	135	139	136	139
Potassium (K)	MMO/L	3.4–4.2	3.9	2.7	3	3.5	3.2	4.3
Chloride (Cl)	MMO/L	96–103	99	96	98	97	96	No result
Enzymes CPK (Creatinine Phospho Kinase)	U/L	< 100	342	358	1216	273	226	233
AST (Aspartate Trans Aminase)	U/L	< 400	448	674	1074	654	529	374
ALP (Alkaline Phosphatase)	U/L	< 180	226	202	209	421	206	229

Table 7   One Blood Sample Laboratory Comparison Exercise

Laboratory comparisons on blood sample from 4 year old mare	Unit	Normal Range	Laboratories		
			A	B	C
Haemoglobin (Hb)	g/L	110–160	183	190	188
Red Cell Count (RCC)	10^{12}/L	7.5–11	9.65	12.7	12.4
Packed Cell Volume (PCV) (HCT)	L/L	0.30–0.48	0.45	0.50	0.48
Mean Corpuscular Volume (MCV) (Red Cells)	fl	41–49	47	39	39
Mean Corpuscular Haemoglobin (MCH)	g/L	13–16	19	15	15
Mean Corpuscular Haemoglobin Concentration (MCHC)	g/L	300–360	400	380	390
Total White Cells (Leucocytes) (WCC)	10^9/L	6–12	9.1	7.8	9.1
Neutrophils	10^9/L	2–7	5.09	5.92	4.82
Basophils	10^9/L	0–0.3	Nil	Nil	0.09
Eosinophils	10^9/L	0.1–0.5	0.18	Nil	0.27
Lymphocytes	10^9/L	1.6–5.4	3.64	1.48	3.64
Monocytes	10^9/L	0.6–0.7	0.18	0.39	0.27
Biochemistry					
Total Plasma Protein (TPP)	g/L	53–76	61	64	62
Sodium (Na)	MMO/L	135–144	136	135	141
Potassium (K)	MMO/L	3.4–4.2	3.2	3.6	3.5
Chloride (Cl)	MMO/L	96–103	96	89	101
Enzymes CPK (Creatinine Phospho Kinase)	U/L	< 100	226	103	205
AST (Aspartate Trans Aminase)	U/L	< 400	529	394	498
ALP (Alkaline Phosphatase)	U/L	< 180	206	385	229

Minerals and Vitamins in the Horse

The health and well-being of the horse, as with humans, depends upon a nutritious well-balanced diet. However, before we can begin to prepare such a diet for our horse, we must have an understanding of the part which minerals and vitamins play in the health of the animal.

We tend to live in a vitamin crazy age and many seem to feel that vitamin supplementation in particular is of paramount importance in every instance. Again, it is easy to fall into the trap that if a little of something is good then more must be better. Healthy horses have been killed by massive over supplementation of vitamin A for example. Post mortems showed massive lesions on the liver, caused by overdosing of this particular vitamin. Few vitamins are dangerous unless grossly overdosed but it is much more sensible to establish positively if there is a specific deficiency in your horse before you waste time and money on supplementation.

In well-managed stables which use only prime fodders, serious vitamin deficiencies are rare. However, this is not quite so true in the case of some minerals, particularly some of the trace minerals. Far too much attention is given today to vitamin supplementation and not enough to certain minerals, which may be deficient. As we have seen earlier in our examination of blood analysis, serious vitamin and/or mineral problems will generally show up somewhere in the blood profile. They may not always be specific but the profile will certainly give us 'clues' which will enable us to further investigate and thus pinpoint a particular deficiency (or toxicity as the case may be).

Minerals

At least 21 minerals are known to be required by the horse in varying degrees. In general terms all of these should be supplied naturally in the diet, when prime fodders are used. However, there is a hidden problem in making this supposition. Just as the horse requires a healthy diet, so the fodders we grow (hays, oats, etc) require a well balanced and properly managed soil to produce healthy crops. Certain soils and certain areas in the world are known to be deficient in certain elements. Naturally crops produced on them may be deficient in such elements, notwithstanding the fact that the crop may grow well and appear to be of excellent quality. Professional farmers will of course be good managers of their land and will take the trouble to judge the quality of their soil. Various government departments of agriculture around the world are well equipped to carry out soil analysis and advise what steps should be taken to bring it up to optimum levels of mineralisation.

Top-dressing with superphosphate (particularly in parts of Australia) has been the 'cure all' for many years, to improve soil quality. However, as with anything overdone, this can inhibit the uptake of calcium, magnesium, cobalt, selenium and copper.

There is an interesting anecdote worth relating here. The trace mineral selenium is important in small doses but it is highly toxic in excessive quantities and selenium toxicity will result in serious hoof problems such as hoof horn separation from the laminae in horses. The story of General Custer's Last Stand, in the early days of US history, is well known. Historians related that a troop of cavalry was on the way to relieve the hard-pressed General. However, their horses were let out to graze on open country, en route for the battle. The native grasses in that particular area contained hugely excessive quantities of selenium.

The result was that all the horses suffered chronic hoof problems within a very short time, so bad that it is believed that the actual horn separated from the laminae of the foot. No doubt the horses had to be put down. As a result, the cavalry did not turn up and history records the fate of General Custer.

The *major* minerals are: *calcium, phosphorus, magnesium, sodium, chlorine, potassium* and *sulphur.*

The *trace* minerals are: *cobalt, copper, fluorine, iodine, iron, manganese, selenium* and *zinc.*

Calcium, phosphorus, magnesium   In horses, a correct balance of calcium, phosphorus and magnesium is absolutely essential. It has been shown that an excess of calcium will cause magnesium to be depleted and vice versa. For this reason, it is probably wiser to supplement dolomite rather than calcium carbonate. In this way the horse will receive some magnesium as well as calcium, which safeguards against magnesium depletion by excess calcium. (By the way, check the purity of any commercial dolomite.)

The calcium/phosphorus balance is also very important. The accepted ratio in the horse is at least 1.5:1 calcium to phosphorus. However, some nutritionists recommend as high as 4:1. The popular cereal feeds and also some hays are quite high in phosphorus but low by comparison in calcium. Good quality lucerne hay (alfalfa), however, has a better balance, being higher in calcium than phosphorus.

Calcium, phosphorus and magnesium are very important in the growth and health of hard tissue. Bone, particularly in young horses and hard working horses (such as race horses), require adequate quantities of these three minerals for healthy skeletal well-being. Magnesium is also vital, as it is the activator of a number of enzymes. Remember that calcium cannot be taken up and used by the system if magnesium is missing or low in the diet.

Severe magnesium deficiency would produce convulsions, sweating and leg swelling. Most prime hays and grains (provided they are grown on the right soils, as already referred to)

Severe calcium deficiency

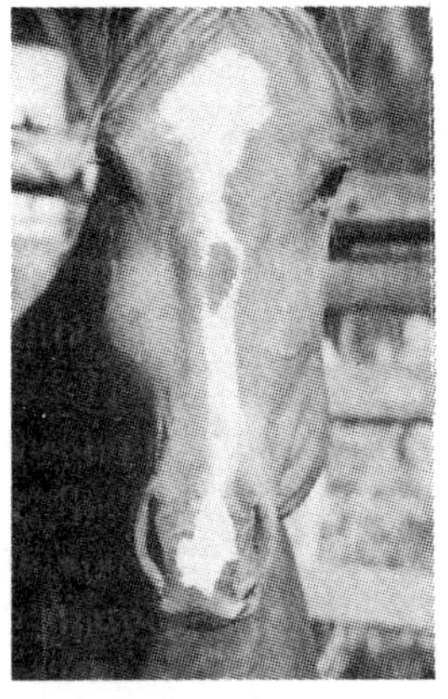

Swelling of the upper jaws (maxillae) from big-head in a horse grazed on buffel grass. The swellings are firm, being composed of the remains of the bone and a large quantity of fibrous tissue. Emerald district, Queensland, 1975.

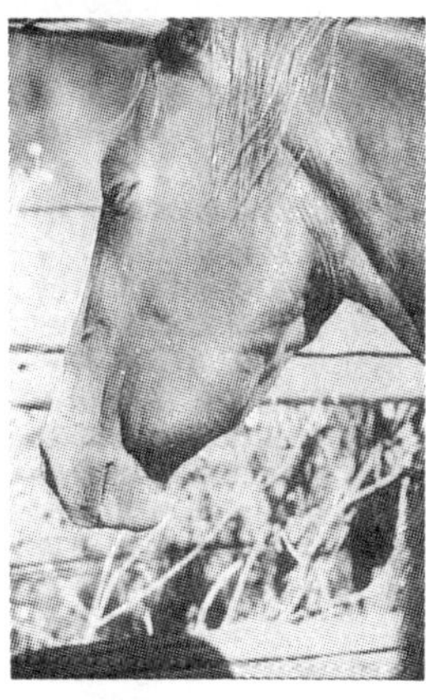

Swelling of the lower jaw (mandible).

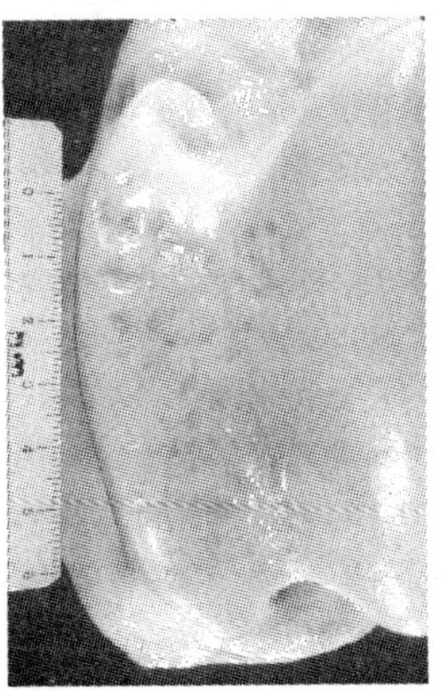

Pitting of the joint surface of a stifle joint in a horse with big-head. Experimental case. The bone supporting the joint has been partly removed by the disease process causing the cartilage covering to collapse. This abnormality is probably associated with lameness seen in this disease.

would contain sufficient magnesium for good nutrition. However, because it is so important, daily supplementation of powdered dolomite (probably about one tablespoonful per day) is essential. The use of a reputable proprietary mineral supplement is strongly recommended. It will supply the full mineral requirements on a daily basis and will take the guesswork out of feeding individual minerals.

As a matter of interest, at this point it is worth comparing the average phosphorus/calcium ratios in some common cereals. *Oats* show approximately 4:1 phosphorus to calcium; *maize* 15:1; *barley* 7:1; *wheat bran* 7:1. This may be quite surprising to some readers because we have already seen that, ideally, we should have at least the *reverse ratio of 1.5:1 calcium to phosphorus*. Again this underlines the advisability of supplementing daily with minerals to ensure adequate calcium/magnesium uptake and other essential minerals.

Wheat bran is a very popular feed used by many horse people daily, in relatively large quantities. In fact it should be regarded as a highly *undesirable* item because it is *very* high in phosphorus and singularly lacking in any meaningful nutritional benefits. It can also chemically bind calcium and therefore prevent its absorption by the horse.

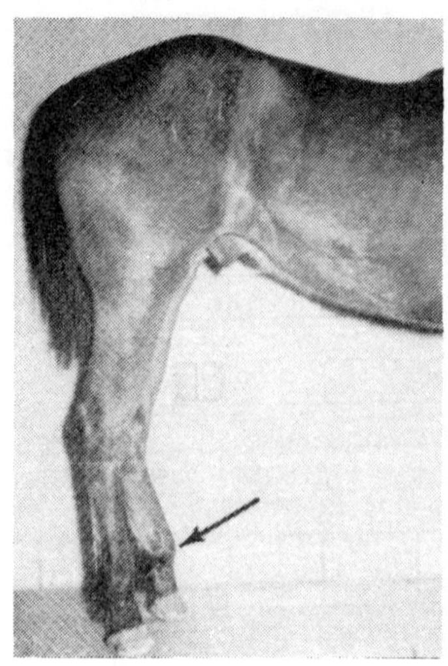

An example of knuckling of the rear fetlocks due to mineral imbalance (rickets).

Having covered the major elements *calcium, phosphorus* and *magnesium*, we shall now examine the remaining four — *sodium, chlorine, potassium* and *sulphur.*

Sodium, chlorine   Sodium and chlorine combined constitute salt (NaCl) as we know it. Salt is important in the acid-base balance and water distribution. Salt deficiency would manifest itself in deprived appetite, rough coat and reduced growth. Na is the principal ion in the extra cellular fluid (ECF), responsible for approximately 50% of the osmosis (tendency of solvent to diffuse through porous partition into more concentrated solution) of the ECF. It can move rapidly between the ECF although its entry into cells is slow. However, concentration of Na within cells can change quickly, due to movement of water into and out of cells.

Most authorities suggest a daily salt intake of 50/60 grams but may be more during heavy sweat loss and in hot climates.

Potassium   This mineral is essential to life. It is a cellular constituent. It assists pressure regulation in the cells and acid balance. If deficient the transmission of nerve impulses would be affected and muscular weakness and paralysis would develop. Hard-working horses can lose significant amounts of potassium (K) in sweat. (We noticed this particularly in our blood testing.) Also the correct potassium level must be maintained for proper heart function. Approximately 98% of body K is in intracellular fluid. For this reason it is thought that plasma/serum K may not always be a reliable guide to total body K.

It is believed that potassium is being lost world-wide due to chemical fertilisers. By their action, they raise the sodium in the soil and potassium is depleted as a result. Because of high sodium levels in many soils, the resulting feed crops are higher in sodium than they should be. It is therefore highly desirable that potassium chloride (KCl) should be available in performance horses.

Sulphur Sulphur is probably being suppressed due to modern farming methods by application of triple superphosphate. It is thought that it may no longer be coming through the food chain. To date there does not appear to have been much in-depth study undertaken of sulphur in relation to equine nutrition. There is no doubt it is essential, but in very small quantities. It is highly toxic in large doses. It was always thought to have been sufficient in most crops to satisfy the daily needs of the equine.

However, we have seen that this may no longer be the case. Lack of sulphur is thought to interfere with the action of some essential amino acids. As a consequence, digestion can be impaired. Skin troubles can be a sign of deficiency. Lice, for example, have been eradicated by sulphur supplementation (as noted by Pat Coleby, a noted Australian authority on animal mineral and vitamin requirements). However, be very careful with this one! Consult your veterinary surgeon before you supplement and be sure that sulphur deficiency is the problem. All minerals are of course inorganic, and are found in the body in pure form and in combination with organic substances. Firstly, they are the *building* substances and secondly, the catalysts in structural elements in body compounds, such as vitamins. They are particularly evident in the hard tissues, bones and teeth in chemical reactions in the formation of these tissues.

In concluding the section on minerals, the words 'major' and 'trace' are used not because of the importance of either category but because of the amounts that are required. The *major* minerals are needed in larger amounts by the horse but the *trace* group minerals only in minute quantities. Measurement of *trace* minerals is usually expressed in milligrams per kilogram or parts per million (PPM).

Now we shall examine the role of the trace minerals: *cobalt, copper, fluorine, iodine, iron, manganese, selenium* and *zinc*.

Cobalt This is a component of the vitamin B12. Deficiency is probably rare, as one would expect all normal feeds to supply the small amount necessary.

Supplementation should only be undertaken on veterinary advice, as it is extremely toxic. It is required for growth and healthy bone development but, although it is essential, cobalt depletion can be considered rare.

Copper   The daily equine requirement has been estimated to be 5–8 PPM. It is essential for bone formation, cartilage and elastin formation, hair pigment and iron utilisation. It is therefore a very important trace element. Deficiency could result in *blood vessel rupture*, brittle bones and anaemia. As we have already noted in the blood analysis section, anaemia is a symptom, not a disease. Iron is mistakenly identified as the cure-all for any form of anaemia. (Note the proliferation of proprietary iron 'tonics' on the market.) However, when *copper is deficient*, *iron cannot be utilised* by the system, so copper deficiency can well be the cause of what many might consider 'iron deficiency'. There also may be some link between copper deficiency and 'bleeding'.

Once again, as with most trace elements, excess copper supplementation is highly toxic. It has also been observed that lack of copper is very likely a reason for horses chewing fences, posts etc. This is not conclusive but some researchers, such as Pat Coleby, have found that a half teaspoon of copper sulphate added daily to the ration has cured persistent fence chewers. Once again, it must be stressed, *proceed with caution*. Be certain that copper deficiency is proven before supplementation of copper sulphate. Veterinary consultation is advised before proceeding.

Fluorine   Fluorine deficiency has not been demonstrated in the horse. However, it should be noted that fluorine over 60 PPM is toxic.

Iodine   This is an essential element for reproduction and physiological processes. It is a compound of the hormone *thyroxine*, which is produced in the thyroid gland. Thyroxine has an influence in almost every body organ — metabolic rate, oxygen consumption, glucose utilisation and protein synthesis. Deficiency may cause enlarged thyroid glands. Iodine deficient feeding to mares can cause weak or stillborn foals. Seaweed meal, routinely fed, should supply all the iodine requirements of the horse.

Iron We have already noted the importance of copper for iron utilisation. Provided this requirement is met, iron deficiency is rare indeed. It is a constituent of haemoglobin, so obviously it is important. However, daily maintenance requirement is probably less than 40 PPM. When we consider that grains alone generally contain 200/400 PPM, it is obvious that horses, properly fed, have literally iron to burn. Notwithstanding this, however, low haemoglobin and packed cell volume levels in racehorses can indicate low iron levels, and supplementation may be required. Stress can depress iron levels.

Manganese Required for enzymes needed in cartilage formation, deficiency may show up in shortened and crooked limbs, and can also contribute to deafness, because of poor development of the cores of the inner ear. The amount has not been defined as yet, but for the horse is thought to be about 40 PPM. Again, it is generally available from normal diet.

Selenium Selenium toxicity is much more widely documented than are its benefits to the horse. As previously mentioned, toxicity manifests itself in hoof and foot problems and is generally caused by horses feeding on pasture growing on seleniferous soils. However, in the 1950s, it was discovered that selenium was shown to prevent white muscle disease. It has also been linked with 'tying up', if not present. It is certain that selenium and vitamin E are vitally involved in healthy muscle growth. Both vitamin E and selenium are anti-oxidants.

As previously mentioned it is highly toxic in excess and caution should be exercised.

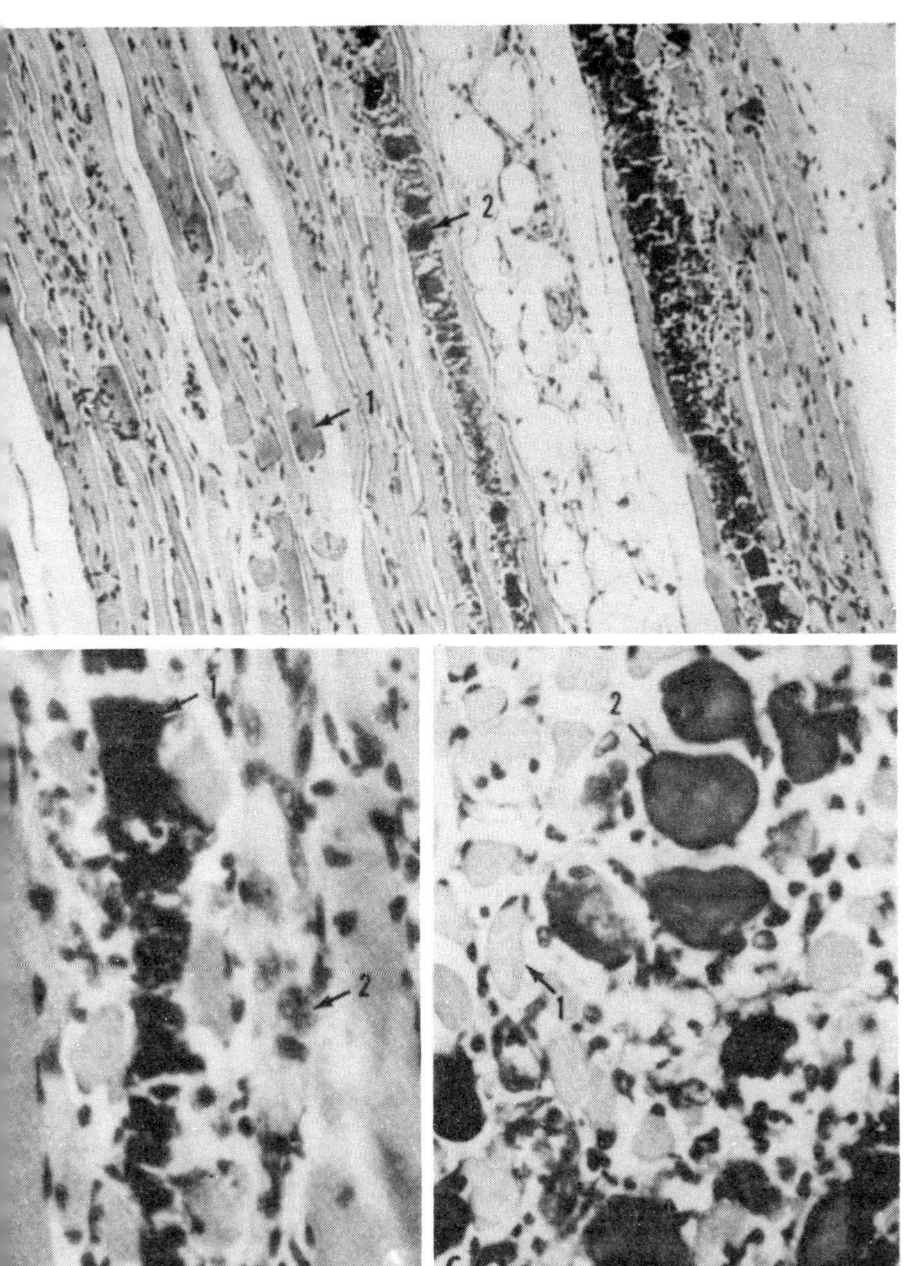

Nutritional myopathy, white-muscle disease, in the tongue of a newborn foal. A, low power (x 150) to show fragmentation of muscle bundles (1) and calcification (2). B, longtitudinal section (x 500) of muscle bundles; calcification within muscle bundles (1), proliferation of sarcolemmal nuclei (2). C, cross section of muscle fibres (x 500); note normal (1) and calcified (2) muscle bundles.

Zinc   The daily zinc requirement is probably less than 5 PPM. Deficiency would show itself in poor growth and skin lesions. It is found in high concentrations in skin and hair but also occurs in bone, muscle, blood and internal organs. Adequate zinc is thought to be available in normal rations.

Incidentally, seaweed meal (provided one can be sure that it has originally come from unpolluted waters) is an excellent and digestible source of many trace elements such as sulphur, cobalt, iodine, selenium and possibly also copper. There are a few good trace mineral supplements on the market; however, many of them leave much to be desired. Carefully check the analysis on the product. Many claiming to be mineral supplements omit important elements such as selenium and zinc but many contain a host of unnecessary elements such as iron.

The importance of water, although not a mineral, should be noted. It is essential to all life as we know and it is vital in digestion, body temperature control and as a solvent. It helps lubricate joints, transmits sound and is required for sight. It must be freely available to the horse at all times. It must always be clean, fresh, without salt and non-fluoridated if possible.

Vitamins

Vitamins are carbon-containing compounds necessary for life and growth. Many cannot be manufactured in sufficient quantities by the body and therefore must be contained in the diet. Vitamins are in two groups — those which are water soluble and those which are fat soluble.

FAT SOLUBLE		WATER SOLUBLE	
Vitamin A	Carotene	B1	Thiamine
Vitamin D		B2	Riboflavin
Vitamin E	Tocopherol	B3	Niacin
Vitamin K	Menadione	B6	Pyridoxine
		B5	Pantothenic Acid
		M	Folic Acid

B12 Cyanocobalamine
      (cobalt is a component of B12)
H   Biotin
–   Choline
C   Ascorbic Acid
–   Inositol
–   PABA

The *water soluble* vitamins are found in their true form in plants and do not require any conversion by the horse's body. The *fat soluble* vitamins are present as provitamins or precursors. These are related substances, which do not have vitamin

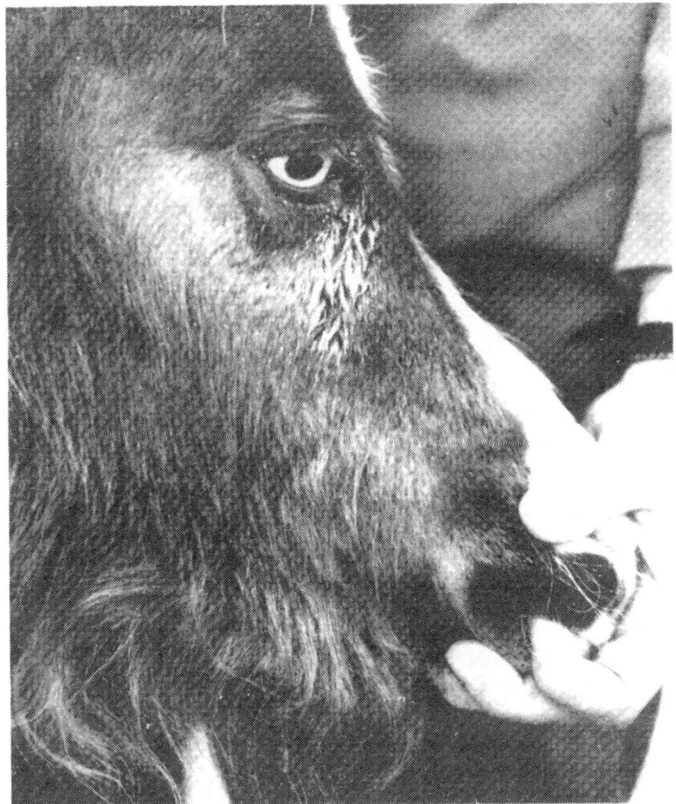

Vitamin A deficiency in a foal - note lacrimation.

action but which are acted upon by the horse's body to yield true vitamins (active form).

Vitamin A   Its primary source in a horse is via its provitamin, the yellow pigment carotene. It is necessary for skin, hair, hooves, eye function. Deficiency would be seen in night blindness, infertility, poor hoof growth, *digestive* and *respiratory problems*. Good green, well-saved, quality lucerne hay would normally supply the vitamin A requirements. Supplementary vitamin A is thought to be around 12,500 international units. Supplementary vitamin A is thought to be beneficial during late pregnancy or heavy training. As mentioned previously, excessive vitamin A can cause liver damage.

Vitamin D   Required for calcium-binding protein formation, this vitamin aids in absorption of calcium/phosphorus. Deficiency could result in rickets, swollen joints, stiffness and reduced serum calcium and phosphorus levels. It is usually supplied to the horse by exposure to sunlight, probably about 20 minutes per day, but can be toxic in excess levels. Some plants like jessamine in the USA can cause such toxicity. Supplementation in cold climates, or during reduced winter sunshine months, may be advisable.

Vitamin E   Necessary for normal cell structure, deficiency can cause a range of problems, such as white muscle disease in foals. It has also recently been discovered that in humans it is vital in the development of the nervous system in early life. It is fairly certain that the same would apply in the equine. It is also thought, in some quarters, to improve fertility in both mares and stallions. Nervous horses have been found to quieten down when supplemented with vitamin E. This would seem to support the link with the development of the nervous system.

Good quality hays contain 50–90 IU per kg. The recommended requirement is thought to be about 15 IU per kg. Wheatgerm and wheatgerm oil are other good sources. Because of its role and importance in nerve health and development, and also its important link with selenium, it is probably one of the few vitamins which should be supplemented regularly. Iron tonics, because they are oxidants, cannot be fed at the same time as vitamin E. They can only be fed at alternative times.

Vitamin K This vitamin is required in the blood clotting process. Internal haemorrhage could result from a deficiency, but is rare in horses, because of the production of significant amounts of vitamin K by bacteria in the intestinal tract.

B Complex B1 (thiamine) Thought to be one of the B group most likely to be missing in horses, thiamine is needed for energy, especially carbohydrate utilisation. Racehorses seem to be prone to a deficiency, because they burn up so much energy. Thiamine injections are sometimes used for 'tying up'. B complex are usually supplied in adequate amounts by good quality hay and/or pasture and also by vitamins produced by bacteria in the gut. Nervous horses often respond to B group supplementation. B1 also stimulates appetite.

B2 (riboflavin) Also involved in energy metabolism, again, hay and pasture may provide adequate amounts.

B12 This is a unique vitamin, not contained in any plants, and contains cobalt. It is required for normal reproduction of red blood cells. Deficiency can cause anaemia and reduced performance. It is produced by bacterial action in the cecum and large intestine if cobalt is present. Weak foals have been found to respond quickly when 10CC of B12 have been injected intramuscularly. Also horses off feed have responded quickly by 20CC B12 injection.

M Folic Acid Again, this is a red blood cell forming vitamin. Good pasture, once again, is an excellent source. Most probably the horse receives sufficient in a balanced diet. Obviously red cell deficiency could point to folic acid shortage. There is no certain knowledge as to the actual level required by the horse. However, we do know it is essential and should be present in all good iron supplements.

B3 Niacin Deficiency is not a problem in horses fed a good balanced ration. Forages and protein supplements (rarely required) are good sources. Recently it has been used to alleviate and help control arthritis and chilblains in humans. It might well have a similar role in the horse. Other than that, B3 has not been identified as playing any particular role in the equine.

B5 Pantothenic Acid This is part of the component of co enzyme A, which is utilised in the metabolism of fat. Like niacin, its function in the horse has not been demonstrated.

B6 Pyridoxine Concerned with protein metabolism, it is possibly needed for resistance to infections, particularly herpes types. (It also plays a part in controlling human travel sickness.) Its role in the horse has not been demonstrated with any certainty.

Biotin This is a B group vitamin which has only gained prominence in recent times. Sources would be seaweed meal, maize and beans. Biotin on its own is available as a feed supplement today. It is thought that in some cases it may play a significant role in recovery from laminitis. It is essential for healthy hoof growth.

Choline Deficiencies have not been reported in horses, so it may be ignored.

Vitamin C Horses, like most animals (humans, guinea pigs and some monkeys being the exceptions) synthesise their own vitamin C requirements in the gut. Until fairly recently, its role in the horse was not understood. However, it now appears to have many functions. It is thought to be essential for healthy cells, for the health and strength of blood vessels and for collagen. It contains lesperidine, which would seem to strengthen blood vessels and it has been used regularly in the treatment of horses prone to break blood vessels under stress (not, of course, the serious pulmonary haemorrhage). It has been used as emergency treatment of snakebite in horses, quite successfully, when antivenene has not been available. Both of these functions of vitamin C administration have been noted by Pat Coleby.

Some little time ago, researchers in Germany found that vitamin C supplementation resulted in horses recovering more quickly from strenuous exercise than those which were not supplemented. Regular routine supplementation of vitamin C would not appear necessary in the healthy horse. However, it does appear to have beneficial effects in many circumstances and it is worth keeping in mind. It also appears to be benign, as far as toxicity is concerned, so it seems fairly safe to experiment with it. Recent tests have also linked it to the immune system. Horses showed markedly lower levels of vitamin C when stressed or suffering viral infections.

However, we have seen that certain trace minerals and vitamins may well be missing, or in short supply even in good fodders. Because of the stress we place on performance horses, and because of fodder quality, there is no doubt that supplementation is of vital importance if we are to optimise the performance of our horses and maintain their good health. A good *mineral supplement* on a daily basis is essential.

The same remarks also apply to a quality *electrolyte*. On the vitamin front, there are one or two good proprietary multivitamins on the market. Specifically, vitamin E (preferably with selenium) and vitamin B1 are the major single vitamin requirements in performance horses.

Select your *brand* of supplements carefully. Read the label and ascertain what you are actually getting for your money. The following advice should be helpful in ensuring that you buy *quality* rather than quantity. Generally speaking the brands produced by veterinary companies are the safest bets. Avoid 'backyard' preparations marketed by firms or individuals who do not employ staff qualified in either veterinary and/or nutritional science.

Don't waste money on 'shotgun' formulations which claim to be the complete answer to all the horse's daily requirements, of both minerals and vitamins. Just like humans, every individual does *not* require supplementation of *every* vitamin and *every* mineral every day. Mineral and vitamin requirements are very different categories. Ascertain what your horse's individual needs are and feed accordingly. Feeding so called 'complete' mixtures is a waste of money and they are very inefficient. They cannot be anything else! Once again, it cannot be over-stressed, *read the label and analysis* carefully before you buy. One well-known electrolyte currently on the Australian market has only 75% active ingredients in the formulation! The balance is a non-active 'filler'. What does this mean? Well, firstly, you are getting only 75% of what you pay for! Secondly, you have to feed at least 33.33% more, by volume, to get the desired result. There are numerous products on the market which fall into this category. On the subject of non-active fillers, there is a legitimate role for them in *certain* formulations and most manufacturers use them. For example, some vitamin B1-based supplements may add a filler like Dextrose to improve the overall palatability. B1 is extremely bitter and many horses, as a result, might refuse the feed to which it has been added.

Certain iron-based preparations may have non-active fillers included, to reduce the concentration of the product. Without a filler, there could be a danger of over-feeding, because such small measures would have to be used to ensure the correct dosage.

However, in general terms, the following types of supplements should *never* include non-active fillers:

Protein (Amino Acid) supplements
Mineral supplements
Carbohydrate boosters

    Single vitamins, such as vitamin E, vitamin C

    Electrolytes

Don't buy 'gimmicky' formulations such as mineral supplement with 'added' vitamin B or 'added' vitamin C. Vitamins cost money and your horse certainly does *not* require an expensive 'added' vitamin each time you administer its mineral supplement. Beware of electrolytes with 'added' vitamins! The 'additions' are *not* body salts (electrolytes) and they have no bodily function in that area to perform. You will pay dearly for them and waste your money as a result.

Make sure that the products are *concentrated* and not 'padded' with non-active fillers as mentioned above. Remember the cost per kilo may look attractive but if you have to feed two or three times the amount, because of the non-active ingredient, then you have been tricked into buying a very expensive formulation. That is why certain manufacturers add them.

When buying electrolytes (apart from the 'fillers' mentioned above and 'bonus' additives), ensure that formulations include the *essential* body salts such as Potassium, Citrate, Sodium Bicarbonate, Sodium Chloride, Magnesium, etc. When buying mineral supplements, make sure that the formulation is a *mineral* formulation *without* vitamins. Check that you have at least a 3:1 ratio Calcium to Phosphorus and that Magnesium is present. Also ensure that all the essential trace elements are there.

Never buy any preparation which contains *both* vitamin E and Iron. They are antagonists, which we have already pointed out. Believe it or not, there are some 'shotgun' preparations on the market which contain both!

Lastly but by no means of less importance, a word on *injectible* supplements. Injections of any sort are best left to the professionals. In unskilled or semi-skilled hands they can be extremely dangerous and sometimes lethal. Depending on what is being injected, the substance is delivered to the animal by three methods: subcutaneous (under the skin), intra-muscular (directly into the muscle) or intravenous (directly into the bloodstream). The latter is potentially the most dangerous, because the dose is delivered almost instantly to the system. There have been cases of horses dropping dead from iron compounds given intravenously. Vitamin and mineral supplements supplied in the food are *infinitely safer*, cheaper, and often more effective. Some individuals excrete injected products more quickly than those ingested by way of food. As a consequence they may not be utilised as efficiently by the system.

In conclusion, your healthy horse needs only good quality fodders, and regular mineral and electrolyte supplements with some regular vitamin supplements. Never be afraid to ask questions and be prepared to learn. There is nothing to be ashamed of in not knowing, but there is something to be ashamed of in not wanting to know. Unfortunately there is a significant number of horse people who seem to believe they know it all.

Bibliography

Agriculture and Equine Diploma Course Notes, Riverina Murray Institute of Higher Education (now Charles Sturt University)

Biochemical Parameters, D.W. Milne, paper presented to the Equine Trauma Centre, New Jersey

Blood Tests, Dr John Kohnke, Australian Horse & Rider

Calcium Deficient Pastures, Dr Ross McKenzie, Queensland Department of Primary Industries, notes

Changes in Haematology Associated with Exercise and Training, Professor R.J. Rose, University of Sydney, paper

Haematology of the Racing Thoroughbred, M. Revington, *Equine Veterinary Journal*

Haematological Responses to Racing and Training, Drs D.H. Sknow (Glasgow), S.W. Ricketts (Newmarket) and D.K. Mason (Hong Kong), *Equine Veterinary Journal*

Horse Nutrition, A Practical Guide, Professor Harold Hintz, PhD, Arco Publishing Inc, New York

Lameness in Horses, O.R. Adams, Lea & Febiger, Philadelphia

Natural Horse Care, Pat Coleby, Night Owl Publishers Pty Ltd, Euroa

Osteodystrophia Fibrosa in Horse at Pasture, Drs Ross McKenzie and J.C. Walthall, Queensland Department of Primary Industries, notes

Veterinary Pathology, T.C. Jones and R.O. Hunt, Lea & Febiger, Philadelphia